SANDRA S. STAFFORD

CONQUERING CHEMOTHERAPY

How to prepare, What's in Store, and How to Overcome Chemotherapy

Contents

Introduction

What is Chemotherapy?

A sound body continually replaces cells through a course of isolating, developing and kicking the bucket. At the point when disease happens, cells repeat wildly and don't pass on when they ought to.

As a piece of the body delivers increasingly more of these unusual cells, they begin to consume the space that valuable cells recently took up.

Chemotherapy drugs disrupt a malignant growth cell's capacity to partition and repeat. Drugs shift by the way they work. Various medications assault malignant growth cells at various stages in the cell life cycle.

Therapy can go after quickly partitioning cells all through the body or just unambiguous substances or portions of malignant growth cells.

In a chemotherapy treatment, a specialist might give an individual a solitary medication or a mix of medications all at once.

What do you want to be familiar with in chemotherapy

Chemotherapy is a therapy that utilizations medicates that kill quickly separating disease cells to keep them from developing and making more cells.

Numerous chemotherapy drugs have antagonistic impacts that can be extreme. Nonetheless, assuming a specialist suggests an individual have chemotherapy, this generally implies that the advantages are probably going to offset any unfriendly impacts.

A singular will frequently go through chemotherapy as a component of a general therapy plan, which may likewise incorporate a medical procedure and radiation treatment. These therapies are powerful in many instances of disease. Notwithstanding, their adequacy will frequently rely upon the sort and phase of malignant growth, among different variables.

Chatting with a specialist will assist an individual with understanding what's in store from chemotherapy.

Peruse on to figure out more about chemotherapy and what it includes.

Chemotherapy can set off a large group of incidental effects, including dry mouth, taste changes, weakness, mouth wounds, and sickness. These can make eating troublesome or unappealing.

Understanding what food varieties to eat, like dull food sources for mouth injuries and wet or velvety surfaces for dry mouth, may assist with sustaining your body while exploring disease treatment.

It's profitable to pack nutritious, go cordial food sources to your arrangements. Rehearsing food handling is likewise critical to bring down your gamble of food contamination.

What do you want to be familiar with in chemotherapy

Chemotherapy is a therapy that utilizations tranquilizers that kill quickly separating disease cells to keep them from developing and making more cells.

Numerous chemotherapy drugs have unfriendly impacts that can be extreme. In any case, assuming that a specialist suggests an individual have chemotherapy, this generally implies that the advantages are probably going to offset any unfriendly impacts.

A singular will frequently go through chemotherapy as a component of a general therapy plan, which may likewise incorporate a medical procedure and radiation treatment. These therapies are successful in many instances of disease. Notwithstanding, their viability will frequently rely upon the sort and phase of the disease, among different variables.

Conversing with a specialist will assist an individual with understanding what's in store from chemotherapy.

What's in store when having Chemotherapy

Chemotherapy is an intrusive treatment that can have serious unfavorable impacts both during the treatment and, surprisingly, later. This is because the medications can't separate between sound and disease cells and will quite often target both.

Nonetheless, people with particular kinds of disease who get early chemotherapy treatment might accomplish a total fix. This makes the secondary effects beneficial for some. Likewise, the vast majority of the undesirable side effects disappear after treatment wraps up.

Getting chemotherapy can be troublesome, and individuals with malignant growth have wretchedness.

An investigation discovered that burdensome side effects are normal in individuals going through chemotherapy and that conjugal and family support assist with dealing with these side effects.

A few people might find it supportive to consult with a guide about the psychological and close-to-home parts of disease and chemotherapy.

It is typical to feel stressed or overpowered when you figure out that you want chemotherapy. Notwithstanding, getting familiar with this sort of disease treatment might assist you with feeling more ready and less restless.

Types of chemotherapy

Kinds of chemotherapy include:

• **Alkylating specialists:** These influence the DNA and kill the cells at various phases of the cell life cycle.

• **Antimetabolites:** These copy proteins that the cells need to make due. At the point when the cells consume them, they offer no advantage, and the cells starve.

• **Plant alkaloids:** These prevent the cells from developing and partitioning.

• **Hostile to growth anti-infection agents:** These prevent the cells from duplicating. They are not the same as the anti-microbials individuals use for diseases.

There is a wide range of classes of medicine that specialists use related to chemotherapy, including monoclonal antibodies, immunotherapy, and designated drugs.

A specialist will suggest a reasonable choice for a person. They might suggest consolidating chemotherapy with different choices, like radiation treatment or medical procedure

Who is in my chemotherapy group?

A profoundly prepared clinical group will cooperate to give you the most ideal consideration. Your group might incorporate these medical services experts:

Clinical oncologist: This kind of specialist has some expertise in treating disease with prescription. Your clinical oncologist works intimately with other colleagues to make your general malignant growth treatment plan. They additionally lead your chemotherapy medicines.

High-level suppliers, similar to oncology nurture specialists (NPS) and oncology doctor colleagues (PAs). These suppliers meet with patients and team up with an overseeing clinical oncologist. Their obligations can include:

• Giving actual assessments

• Requesting and deciphering research center and symptomatic experimental outcomes

• Recommending and overseeing drugs and different treatments, including chemotherapy

• Giving training and directing to patients and families

Oncology nurture: Oncology nurture works in malignant growth care. This incorporates giving chemotherapy. Oncology medical caretakers can likewise:

• Answer inquiries regarding treatment

• Screen your wellbeing during treatment

• Assist you with overseeing the results of treatment

Other medical services experts. Other colleagues might help care for your physical, profound, and social necessities during chemotherapy. These experts include:

- **Drug specialists**
- **Social specialists**
- **Enrolled dietitian nutritionists**
- **Actual advisors**
- **Dental specialists**

What occurs before chemotherapy?

Every chemotherapy treatment plan is made to meet a patient's remarkable requirements. Be that as it may, before treatment begins, you can hope to make these general strides.

Meet with your oncologist: The specialist will investigate your clinical records and do an actual test. You will likewise have tests done to assist with arranging treatment. Your definite therapy relies upon the kind, size, and area of the disease. Your primary care physician will likewise think about your age, your overall wellbeing, and different elements, like past disease medicines.

Find out about your chemotherapy therapy plan: Your medical services group will make sense of when and how frequently you want chemotherapy. Most chemotherapy medicines are given in rehashing cycles. The length of a cycle relies upon the drug(s) you get. Most cycles range from 2 to about a month and a half. The quantity of therapy portions booked inside each cycle likewise relies upon the recommended chemotherapy.

For instance, each cycle might contain just 1 portion right off the bat: Or on the other hand, a cycle might contain more than 1 portion given every week or every day. Frequently, your PCP will check assuming that the treatment is working after you finish 2 cycles. The vast majority have a few patterns of chemotherapy. In some cases, chemotherapy treatment is progressing as an upkeep treatment.

Give authorization for chemotherapy: Your primary care physician will talk with you about the potential dangers and advantages of chemotherapy. This conversation will incorporate likely momentary aftereffects and late impacts of the chemotherapy. This is an extraordinary time for you to get clarification on pressing issues and offer any worries. When you choose to push ahead, your medical services group will request that you sign an educated assent structure.

Marking this structure implies:

· Your group gave you data on your treatment choices.

· You decide to have chemotherapy.

· You give consent for medical services experts to convey the therapy.

· You comprehend that the treatment isn't ensured to give the expected outcomes.

· You comprehend that there are potential dangers, similar to incidental effects, that might occur because of the treatment.

Your medical care group will let you know if there are limitations or ideas about what to eat and drink on chemotherapy days. This will assist your treatment with working best. Continuously tell your chemotherapy group about any remedy and non-professionally prescribed meds you take. Incorporate nutrients and different enhancements, like spices. This is to keep away from drug connections and other undesirable incidental effects. Your primary care physician will let you know if you shouldn't accept them during chemotherapy.

How long does it endure?

The specialist will arrange with a person that indicates when treatment meetings will happen and the number of meetings the singular will that need.

An individual might get chemotherapy for a particular measure of time or however long it works.

A course of chemotherapy therapy normally endures 3-6 months, contingent upon the kind of medication and phase of malignant growth. Specialists normally oversee chemotherapy in cycles, with rest periods between 1 a month. Cycles have to rest in the middle to permit an individual's body to recuperate.

An individual could have treatment on one day, trailed by multi week's rest, then an additional 1-day treatment followed by a 3-week rest period, etc. An individual might rehash this timetable a few times.

Blood tests: Blood tests survey an individual's wellbeing and guarantee that they will want to adapt to conceivable incidental effects.

Liver wellbeing: The liver separates chemotherapy synthetic substances and different medications. Over-burdening the liver could set off different issues. On the off chance that a blood test recognizes liver issues before treatment, an individual might need to defer treatment until the liver recuperates.

Complete blood count: Doctors will take a look at an individual's red platelet (RBC), white platelet (WBC), and platelet count before treatment. If these are low, an individual might have to hold on until they arrive at solid levels before beginning chemotherapy.

It is fundamental to have ordinary blood tests all through the treatment period to guarantee that blood and liver capabilities stay as ideal as could be expected and to screen the adequacy of the treatment.

How could I anticipate chemotherapy medicines?

There are steps you can take before treatment starts to assist you with adapting.

Plan for secondary effects: Your group will work with you to make arrangements for secondary effects normal to your particular treatment. These may incorporate sickness and spewing, weariness, and opposite secondary effects. This can incorporate suggestions about eating great and getting customary activity.

Alleviating physical and close-to-home aftereffects is a significant piece of your general disease treatment: This sort of care is called palliative consideration or steady consideration. Converse with your medical services group about the aftereffects you experience and ways of overseeing and treating them. Dive deeper into the results of chemotherapy.

Make a providing care arrangement: Individuals getting chemotherapy might require additional assistance during treatment with transportation, family errands, and different undertakings. Loved ones can offer a significant help during this time, called providing care. Ask your group what kind of providing care at home you might require during and after treatment.

Find support with funds: Malignant growth treatment can be exorbitant. Before chemotherapy begins, talk with your group about the monetary contemplations of your treatment, including explicit protection inclusion. You might need to contact associations that can offer monetary help. This could be significant on the off chance that your health care coverage doesn't take care of the entire expense of treatment.

Find support at work: As you find out about your therapy timetable and aftereffects, you might be worried about what this could mean for your plan for getting work done. Consult with your boss about potential acclimations to your plan for getting work done or different courses of action during treatment and your recuperation.

How is the portion given?

There are different approaches to taking chemotherapy. These include:

· oral, as tablets, fluid, or cases

· intravenous (IV), as an infusion or mixture into a vein and straightforwardly into the circulation system

· effective, onto the skin

· through an infusion, as a shot in a muscle or right under the skin

· intrathecal, infused into a liquid-occupied space between the tissues covering the mind and the spinal rope, for diseases that arrived at the cerebrospinal liquid

· intraperitoneal, straightforwardly into the peritoneum, or the covering of the outer layer of the mid-region encompassing inward organs, like the stomach and the digestion tracts

· intra-blood vessel, infused to a supply route that goes straightforwardly to the malignant growth

The vast majority will get chemotherapy in a facility or an emergency clinic, yet in some cases, they can take it at home. An individual who gets chemotherapy drugs at home ought to take the portion precisely as recommended. On the off chance that they neglect to take a portion with impeccable timing, they ought to contact their PCP right away.

They will in any case have to make ordinary visits to the medical clinic for specialists to take a look at their wellbeing and reaction to therapy.

An individual getting drugs through an IV gets it through a needle or different instruments, for example,

• **Catheter:** A specialist places one finish of a dainty, delicate cylinder in a huge vein close to the heart, and the opposite end stays outside the body.

• **Port:** Ports are little circles embedded under the skin and stay there until an individual completes their treatment. A catheter interfaces the port to a vein close to the heart through the chest, arm, or midsection.

• **Siphon:** Healthcare experts frequently join these catheters or ports for a more controlled arrival of medications. Siphons can be precisely embedded under the skin or conveyed externally to the body.

What occurs during chemotherapy treatment?

There are various ways you can get chemotherapy. The most widely recognized way that chemotherapy drugs are given is through a needle into a vein. This is called intravenous or IV chemotherapy. Chemotherapy can likewise be taken as a pill, container, or fluid by mouth, as an infusion or shot, or as a cream that is placed straightforwardly on your skin. Get familiar with the various types of chemotherapy.

During your most memorable IV chemotherapy arrangement, you ought to bring a companion or relative: They can uphold you and assist you with recalling data. Some of the time you will be given medicine before your chemotherapy treatment that can make you tired, so you might require somebody who can drive you home.

You may likewise bring things that make your treatment time more straightforward: For example, taking into account bringing your telephone, a tablet, books, or a cover.

Before your treatment begins, you will:

· Have a blood test taken

· Meet with your oncologist so they can check your wellbeing and blood test results

· Meet the medical caretaker or other wellbeing experts who will give your therapy

· Have your circulatory strain, heartbeat, breathing, and temperature taken before beginning treatment

· Have your level and weight estimated to track down the right portion of chemotherapy

· May have an IV cylinder, likewise called a catheter, put in your arm

Certain individuals get chemotherapy through a port: Rather than putting the IV straightforwardly into your arm, the catheter will go into a round metal or plastic plate. With a port, your medical caretaker doesn't have to track down a vein to place the IV in for every therapy. If you want a port, you will require a minor medical procedure before your most memorable chemotherapy arrangement to place the port. Study catheters and ports.

The length of your treatment meeting will rely upon many variables: Some chemotherapy medicines require minutes or hours. Others are allowed north of a few days or weeks. This is called constant implantation chemotherapy. You don't have to remain at the medical clinic or facility for the ceaseless mixture. All things considered, drugs are conveyed through a little siphon you wear or convey.

To get the full advantage of chemotherapy, it is essential to follow the timetable of medicines suggested by your PCP and oversee the different meds you're taking.

What occurs after IV chemotherapy closes?

After your treatment meeting closes, the medical attendant or another medical services colleague will take out your IV. If you have a port, it will remain in until you finish your medicines as a whole. The medical attendant will check your circulatory strain, heartbeat, breathing, and temperature once more.

Your oncologist or attendant will talk with you about what's in store with aftereffects: They will give you medicine, let you know how to oversee normal aftereffects, and proposition data, for example,

• **Stay away from individuals with colds or different contaminations:** Chemotherapy debilitates your body's insusceptible framework. Your insusceptible framework helps battle contaminations.

• **Drink loads of liquids for 48 hours after chemotherapy:** This helps move the medications through your body.

• Whether there are exercises to do or try not to do on future treatment days.

Before you leave your most memorable treatment, make certain to ask who you ought to call with any various forms of feedback and how to reach them, including night-time or end of the week.

Inquiries to pose to the medical services group

• Who is making my chemotherapy treatment plan? How frequently will the arrangement be checked on?

• Which medical care experts will I see at each therapy meeting?

• How might I get chemotherapy medicines? Will I want a port?

• Will I want any tests or sweeps before this treatment starts?

• Could you at any point portray what my most memorable treatment will be like?

• What amount of time will every treatment meeting require?

• Will I want somebody to drive me home after every meeting?

• How frequently will I have chemotherapy? For how long?

• What are the normal symptoms of the chemotherapy I will get?

• Who would it be advisable for me to converse with about any aftereffects I encounter?

• Would it be advisable for me to follow the secondary effects I experience at home?

• Are their secondary effects I ought to tell you about immediately?

• Who might I at any point chat with assuming that I'm having a restless outlook on having this treatment?

• What kind of providing care might I at any point require at home?

• How might we be aware if the chemotherapy is working?

• What follow-up care will I want after chemotherapy?

12 normal incidental effects

Chemotherapy can deliver unfavorable outcomes that reach from gentle to extreme, contingent upon the sort and degree of the treatment. Certain individuals might encounter not many to no antagonistic impacts.

12 normal incidental effects

C hemotherapy can deliver unfavorable outcomes that reach from gentle to extreme, contingent upon the sort and degree of the treatment. Certain individuals might encounter not many to no antagonistic impacts.

Many antagonistic impacts can happen, including:

1. Queasiness and retching: Sickness and retching are run-of-the-mill aftereffects. Specialists might recommend antiemetic medications to assist with lessening the side effects.

Ginger has bioactive mixtures called gingerols and shogaols that have numerous advantages for chemotherapy patients going through treatment.

2. Hair, nails, and skin: Chemotherapy drugs assault quickly developing cells, like hair cells. This might make certain individuals experience going bald or make their hair meager or fragile for half a month in the wake of beginning their treatment.

Wearing cooling covers can keep the scalp cool during chemotherapy treatment, which might help forestall or decrease going bald. Scalp cooling forestalled going bald as well as caused quicker recuperation of hair volume after treatment.

The vast majority find that their hair comes back whenever they have completed treatment. A guide might offer counsel about getting a hairpiece or one more reasonable covering during treatment.

Chemotherapy can likewise influence the skin and nails. Nail changes can include:

• more slender, more fragile nails

- agonizing nail beds
- dry, broken skin in the fingernail skin
- variety changes
- edges or stamps in the nails
- lifting or tumbling off of nails
- slow nail development

The skin might end up being dry and sore. It might likewise become oversensitive to daylight, which medical services experts call photosensitivity. Individuals ought to take care in direct daylight, including:

- keeping away from the sun around early afternoon
- utilizing sunblock
- wearing garments that give the most extreme insurance

3. Weariness: Weariness is among the most incessant symptoms of chemotherapy. An individual might encounter this more often than not or solely after specific exercises.

To lessen weakness, an individual can counsel a specialist about what the right equilibrium between movement and rest is for them. Much of the time, it is ideal to keep away from complete rest except if a specialist has trained it.

Keeping a degree of active work might assist with side effects and may mean an individual can continue with regular day-to-day existence however much as could reasonably be expected.

4. Hearing impedance: The poisons in certain kinds of chemotherapy can influence the sensory system, prompting:

- tinnitus, or ringing in the ears
- transitory or extremely durable hearing misfortune
- balance issues

An individual ought to report any conference changes to the specialist.

5. Diseases: WBCs assist with safeguarding the body from contamination. Chemotherapy can make the quantity of WBCs fall, debilitating the safe framework and expanding the gamble of contaminations.

Individuals ought to play it safe to diminish their probability of getting a disease. These include:

- washing the hands routinely

- keeping any injuries clean
- keeping fitting food cleanliness rules
- seeking early treatment if they suspect a disease
- staying away from contact with individuals who could have an irresistible disease

A specialist might endorse anti-microbials to assist with diminishing the gamble.

People with febrile neutropenia ought to likewise stay away from openness to the soil. They might need to abstain from cultivating, digging, outside development, and comparative exercises.

6. Draining issues: Chemotherapy can lessen an individual's platelet count. This implies the blood will never again clump as successfully.

The individual might have insight:

- simple swelling
- more draining than expected from a little cut
- incessant nosebleeds or draining gums

On the off chance that the platelet count falls too low, an individual might require blood bonding.

Individuals ought to take additional consideration while participating in exercises like cooking, planting, or shaving, to lessen the gamble of harming themselves.

7. Pallor: Chemotherapy can cause RBC levels to fall, which will prompt pallor. Around 70% of individuals going through chemotherapy foster sickliness.

Side effects include:

- sleepiness
- windedness
- heart palpitations

Consuming additional iron might assist the body with making more RBCs. Individuals can take in additional iron from their eating routine. Great food sources include:

- dull green verdant vegetables
- beans

- meat

- nuts

- prunes, raisins, and apricots

Specialists might give blood bondings to individuals encountering extreme or deteriorating side effects of paleness.

8. **Mucositis**: Mucositis, or aggravation of the mucous layer, can influence any piece of the stomach-related framework, from the mouth to the butt.

Oral mucositis influences the mouth. Side effects can differ contingent upon the chemotherapy portion. It can make it difficult to eat or talk, while certain people experience a consuming aggravation in their mouth or all the rage.

In the case of draining happens, it might mean an individual has a disease or is in danger of one. It frequently seems 7-10 Confided in Source days in the wake of beginning treatment and regularly vanishes half a month after treatment.

A specialist might recommend a drug to help forestall or treat it.

9. Loss of craving: Chemotherapy, malignant growth, or both can influence how the body processes supplements, which can prompt a deficiency of hunger and weight reduction.

The seriousness of these secondary effects relies upon the kind of disease and chemotherapy treatment, yet an individual normally recaptures their craving after treatment.

Tips to determine this incorporate eating more modest, more incessant dinners and polishing off supplement-rich beverages, for example, smoothies, through a straw, to assist with keeping up with liquid and supplement consumption.

Individuals who find it excessively challenging to eat ought to talk with a specialist for counsel.

10. Pregnancy and fruitfulness: Individuals frequently lose interest in sex during chemotherapy, however, they for the most part recover it after treatment.

10a. Ripeness: A few sorts of chemotherapy can decrease an individual's ripeness. Frequently, these profits after treatment are finished. Notwithstanding, individuals who wish to have youngsters in the future might think about freezing sperm or undeveloped organisms for some time in the future.

10b. Pregnancy: Chemotherapy can make serious antagonistic side impacts, and thusly, it could be ideal to abstain from becoming pregnant while having treatment.

A specialist can prompt on reasonable conception prevention techniques. Anybody who is pregnant or becomes pregnant during chemotherapy treatment ought to tell their PCP without a moment's delay.

11. Gut issues: Chemotherapy can likewise prompt the runs or clogging, as the body removes harmed cells. Side effects frequently start a couple of days after treatment begins.

A specialist might endorse drugs to assist with the runs before treatment starts. On the off chance that an individual feels they are becoming dried out because of looseness of the bowels, they ought to contact a specialist immediately.

12. Mental and psychological wellness issues: I found that people who got chemotherapy had more awful mental capability a half year after getting chemotherapy.

Chemotherapy can likewise prompt trouble with thinking, arranging, and performing various tasks. Certain individuals experience a state of mind swings and melancholy.

The actual treatment and an individual's tension about the condition may likewise set off or deteriorate these side effects.

Food to watch during chemotherapy

1. Cereal: Cereal gives various supplements that can help your body during chemo.

It brags adequate sums of carbs, protein, and cancer prevention agents, as well as additional sound fats than most grains. It likewise controls your entrails given its beta-glucan, a sort of dissolvable fiber that takes care of the great microbes in your stomach.

Oats' unbiased flavor and smooth surface are particularly profitable assuming you're encountering normal chemos secondary effects like dry mouth or mouth bruises.

Also, you can take for the time being oats to your chemo arrangements. To make this dish, essentially absorb oats milk of your decision and refrigerate for the time being. Toward the beginning of the day, you can finish off it with berries, honey, or nuts.

On the off chance that you're taking cereal in a hurry, eat it in something like 2 hours to stay away from foodborne diseases — however you can limit this gamble by keeping it in a cooler.

Natural products, maple syrup, and nuts are normal add-ins, however, you can likewise make appetizing oats with avocado or eggs. Eat it plain or with a hint of salt if you're encountering sickness or mouth bruises.

Cereal gives various supplements and is tasteful assuming you're encountering chemo side effects like dry mouth, mouth bruises, and queasiness. Its fiber can likewise assist with keeping your solid discharge standard.

2. Avocado: On the off chance that your craving is deficient with regards to, avocados can pack important calories and supplements into your eating routine.

This velvety, green natural product is especially high in sound monounsaturated fat, which can assist with bringing down LDL (terrible) cholesterol while raising HDL (great) cholesterol. It's additionally stacked with fiber, with 3.5 ounces (100 grams) pressing 27% of the Daily Value (DV).

Its fiber beefs up your stool and feeds the cordial microbes in your stomach.

Since they're filling, flexible, and gentle, avocados are an extraordinary choice if you're encountering dry mouth, clogging, mouth wounds, or weight reduction.

You can crush and spread them on toast or cut them to top a bowl of grains, beans, or soup.

Simply make certain to wash unpeeled avocados before you cut them, as their skin can hold onto Listeria, a typical bacterium that can cause.

Avocados are an additionally healthful force to be reckoned with. With a lot of fat and fiber, they can keep you full and give you the required calories when your hunger is low.

3. Eggs: Exhaustion is a typical result of chemotherapy.

Eggs might battle sluggishness because of their liberal stock of protein and fats — almost 6 grams of protein and 4 grams of fat in a solitary medium-sized egg (44 grams).

While fat furnishes your body with energy, protein keeps up with and fabricates bulk, which is particularly significant during chemotherapy.

You can hard-bubble eggs for a versatile tidbit or scramble them for a flavorful feast. Ensure that they're completely cooked, with thickened yolks and solidified whites, to forestall food contamination.

Their delicate, mitigating surface makes eggs ideal on the off chance that you're encountering mouth wounds.

Eggs might ease weakness because of their mix of protein and fats. Furthermore, they're not difficult to eat assuming you have mouth injuries.

4. Stock: Taste changes are ordinary during chemotherapy — and water is normally said to taste unique.

On these occasions, the stock is an extraordinary choice to keep you hydrated. It's made by stewing water with vegetables, spices, and — whenever wanted

— meat or poultry, in addition to bones.

During this interaction, electrolytes are delivered into the liquid. These charged particles, which incorporate supplements like sodium, potassium, chloride, and calcium, assist with keeping your body working appropriately.

Tasting on stock can be useful assuming you're losing electrolytes through regurgitation, sweat, or looseness of the bowels.

Assuming you have the craving for it, you can add chicken, tofu, or veggies into your stock. Puréeing this blend will assist it with going down more straightforwardly assuming that you have mouth wounds.

For added supplements, particularly while you're encountering dry mouth or low craving, you can stack in a spoonful of flavorless protein powder, for example, collagen powder.

Be that as it may, keep your stock clear and straightforward assuming you're encountering sickness or regurgitating — and taste gradual. Stock is perfect for these occasions, as its absence of fiber makes it more straightforward to process.

Clear stock assists you with remaining hydrated and recharged, particularly assuming that water begins tasting diversely during your chemo. You can add veggies or protein on the off chance that you're feeling ready to deal with strong food.

5. Almonds and different nuts: During chemotherapy, you might wind up all through a lot of arrangements — so tidbits can prove to be useful.

In addition to the fact that nuts are like almonds and cashews simple to take in a hurry, however, they additionally gloat adequate measures of protein, solid fats, nutrients, and minerals.

Almonds are a rich wellspring of manganese and copper, giving 27% and 32% of the DV, individually, per 1 ounce (28 grams).

These minerals structure superoxide dismutases, probably the most remarkable cell reinforcements in the body. Cancer prevention agents assist with battling free revolutionaries that harm your cells.

You can likewise add nuts to oats or different dishes.

Nonetheless, they may be not difficult to eat on the off chance that you're encountering mouth injuries. On these occasions, pick nut spreads all things being equal.

Almonds brag a noteworthy number of supplements, including manganese and copper, and act as an optimal tidbit.

6. Pumpkin seeds: Like nuts, pumpkin seeds are perfect for eating between your arrangements.

They're plentiful in fats, protein, and cell reinforcements like vitamin E, which can assist with battling irritation.

Additionally, they convey almost 3 grams of iron for every 1/3 cup (33 grams) or around 15% of the DV.

In any case, a few medicines, like blood bondings, may expand your gamble of iron over-burden, or overabundance of iron in your body. On the off chance that you foster this condition, you'll need to watch your admission of pumpkin seeds and other high-iron food.

For a sweet-and-pungent contort, make your path blend by joining pumpkin seeds, dried cranberries, and other dried organic products, seeds, and nuts.

Pumpkin seeds are perfect for hurry snacks and are particularly wealthy in solid fats and iron. However, assuming that you have iron over-burden, you might need to restrict your admission.

7. Broccoli and other cruciferous vegetables: Cruciferous vegetables, including kale, broccoli, cauliflower, and cabbage, brag a noteworthy healthful profile.

Specifically, broccoli offers a lot of L-ascorbic acids. This nutrient is crucial for your insusceptible framework.

Furthermore, it contains sulforaphane, a plant compound idea to further develop mind wellbeing.

Research has shown that sulforaphane can decidedly affect mental well-being by diminishing irritation and safeguarding cells from harm, which is particularly significant while going through chemotherapy.

Steam or dish these veggies with olive oil and a smidgen of salt. If you're encountering taste changes, attempt a press of lemon as long as you don't have mouth wounds or sickness.

Broccoli and other cruciferous veggies are high in supplements your body needs. Specifically, broccoli contains sulforaphane, a plant compound that might assist with safeguarding cerebrum wellbeing.

8. Hand-crafted smoothies: Handcrafted smoothies are an extraordinary choice if you're struggling with biting strong food or getting an adequate number of supplements in your eating regimen.

They're exceptionally adjustable, permitting you to pick the best elements for your side effects or taste changes.

Here is an essential smoothie recipe:

• 1-2 cups (240-475 ml) of fluid

• 1.5-3 cups (225-450 grams) of veggies or potentially natural product

• 1 tablespoon (15 grams) of protein

• 1 tablespoon (15 grams) of fat

For example, consolidate new or frozen natural products with milk or kefir, then, at that point, throw in a small bunch or two of washed spinach leaves. Dump in a spoonful of flax seeds for fat and peanut butter for protein.

Assuming that you're utilizing new berries, make certain to splash them before washing them completely in running water. This will assist with eliminating any flotsam and jetsam or microorganisms that could make you wiped out.

You can likewise press in a touch of lemon or lime to light up the flavors.

Smoothies are an extraordinary choice for times when eating is troublesome. Besides, they're an optimal method for adding foods grown from the ground to your eating routine.

9. Bread or saltines: If you're encountering looseness of the bowels or queasiness, white bread or saltines are a decent decision since they're regularly simple to process. Entire grain renditions, which supply added supplements, are great for when your stomach isn't disturbed.

Salted wafers or saltines are particularly valuable to recharge sodium lost through the runs or spewing.

Eat them plain or top with nut spread, crushed avocado, or ricotta cheddar assuming that you want more flavor and supplements.

White bread and wafers can be useful assuming looseness of the bowels or sickness set in. Saltines can assist with reestablishing sodium lost to loose bowels or spewing.

10. Fish: If you appreciate fish, it's smart to eat two servings of fish each week when you're in chemotherapy. That is because it gives protein and omega-3 unsaturated fats.

Omega-3s are significant fats that you should traverse your eating regimen. They support cerebrum wellbeing and brag calming properties. Besides, eating a lot of protein and sound fat-rich food varieties like fish can assist you with staying away from undesirable weight reduction during treatment.

Salmon, mackerel, tuna fish, and sardines are especially high in these fats.

What's fattier fish like salmon and herring is a rich wellspring of vitamin D, which is fundamental for legitimate bone and resistant wellbeing. A little salmon filet (170 grams) gives 113% of the DV.

Steam, sear, or broil your fish with a crush of lemon. Utilize a meat thermometer to be certain it arrives at an inside temperature of something like 145°F (63°C) — or 165°F (74°C) on the off chance that you're warming it.

Fish can be a rich wellspring of omega-3 unsaturated fats and vitamin D. Besides, eating protein and fat-rich food sources like fish high in omega-3s can assist with forestalling undesirable weight reduction, and vitamin D are significant for resistance. Expect to eat two servings each week.

Food sources to avoid during chemotherapy

Assuming you have the disease, you might not have quite a bit of hunger, especially during or after your treatment meetings. Notwithstanding, eating great is essential to assist your body with adapting to both the illness and treatment. What's more, similarly as there are quality food varieties to add to your eating regimen, there are a few food varieties to keep away from malignant growth. A few food varieties might seriously jeopardize you for foodborne disease, or food contamination, while others might cause torment or cause you to feel all the sicker. Converse with your primary care physician about the right nourishment plan during your therapy, however for the most part it's really smart to keep these food sources out of your eating routine assuming you're living with a disease.

1. Unpasteurized Dairy Products: While going through malignant growth treatment, your safe framework can't safeguard you as well to no one's surprise. Unpasteurized dairy items, like crude milk and crude yogurt, and delicate cheeses like Brie, may contain microscopic organisms that could make you wiped out. This incorporates items from cows, sheep, and goats. Typically, your body might have the option to adapt to these microscopic organisms, yet on the off chance that you have a compromised safe framework, you could create an extreme infection.

2. Raw Eggs: Eggs are a convenient, nutritious parcel of food. You can eat them in many structures — bubbled, mixed, broiled — and you can add them to a few dishes. However, stay away from any dish that contains crude or delicately cooked eggs, for example, pasta carbonara or Hollandaise sauce. Eggs that aren't cooked as expected can contain Salmonella microbes, which can cause disease with similar side effects as from polluted dairy items. A well-known method for consuming crude eggs is in smoothies. Smoothies with leafy foods can be solid, however on the off chance that you include a crude egg, you risk making the smoothie hazardous.

3. Unwashed Produce: Always wash the produce you bring back from the store or market, regardless of whether it's named "pre-washed." Be particularly mindful of products of the soil you develop yourself, particularly verdant ones. Soil may not generally be apparent, however, it could contain microorganisms that could make you genuinely sick. This incorporates local or locally acquired new spices, like basil or thyme. On the off chance that a natural product or vegetable has a skin you will not or can't eat, wash it in any case since, in such a case that you slice through the skin with a blade, you could get soil from outside the produce towards the tissue.

4. Undercooked Meat: If you like your cheeseburger intriguing or partake in a periodic steak tartare, stop. Half-cooked meat and poultry, and crude fish, similar to shellfish, may contain microbes or infections that can cause foodborne ailments. The insignificant interior temperature for cuts of meat, pork, veal, and sheep is 145 degrees Fahrenheit. Ground meat ought to be at least 160 degrees. Poultry ought to be 165 degrees, at least, while fish and shellfish ought to be 145 degrees minimum.

5. Raw Vegetable Sprouts: Raw vegetable fledglings are becoming famous in ordinary food. They add a visual pop and perhaps a pleasant smash to a serving of mixed greens, and they truly do have medical advantages. Nonetheless, these fledglings have additionally been liable to reviews throughout the long term, because of tainting. A few kinds of tainting, like E. coli, may not be quickly wiped off the produce, so it is more secure to try not to devour them while your safe framework isn't at its strongest.

6. Hot or Cold Foods that have been left out : Whether it's in your kitchen or you're visiting a companion for a smorgasbord style supper, stay away from food sources that ought to be hot or cold yet have been forgotten about at room temperature for two hours or more. Hot food sources ought to remain at 140 degrees Fahrenheit or higher and cold food varieties ought to be 40 degrees or lower. If you truly do have a smorgasbord, slow cookers (connected!) can keep food warm, as can warming plates and scraping dishes. Ice showers can assist with keeping food cold.

7. Junk Food: If you're out of nowhere eager or you have a desire, unhealthy food might entice you. However, chips and cheap food dinners don't contain the supplements your body needs while you are going through malignant growth treatment. They might top you off for a brief time, however, you might be hungrier all the more rapidly as the food goes through you. Additionally, many quick food varieties are high in salt, which can dry out you. On the off chance that you truly should fulfill a hankering, in any case, do as such with some restraint. A little aiding might be all you want, without upsetting your customary dinners.

8. Foods With Sharp or Spicy Flavors: Potential results of certain sorts of radiation and chemotherapy are bruises in your mouth, an irritated throat, and sickness and retching. Keep away from any food sources or beverages that are acrid, tart, acidic, or zesty, as these may make the wounds more difficult. All things considered, pick tasteless choices, for example, cream–based soups, pudding, milkshakes, or cooked or canned leafy foods. Emphatically enhanced food varieties can likewise set off a sickness or exacerbate it. It can take experimentation to find the food varieties that turn out best for you.

9. Food and Drinks that are Dehydrating: While you are getting disease treatment, it's critical to remain hydrated. Assuming you eat or drink something that is drying out, this could make the incidental effects more articulated. Avoid feasts that are exceptionally pungent, and stay away from drinks with liquor or caffeine, as they are additionally drying out. If you're extremely parched, it very well might be enticing to go after anything, including a cola. All things being equal, hydrate consistently over the day to extinguish your thirst before it begins.

Care for your body after treatment

Straightforward advances can work on your feeling of prosperity and your satisfaction after malignant growth treatment. Figure out what you can do.

After your disease therapy, as a malignant growth survivor, you're anxious to get back to great wellbeing. However, past your underlying recuperation, there are ways of further developing you're drawn-out well-being with the goal that you can partake in the years ahead as a disease survivor.

The proposals for disease survivors are the same as the suggestions for any individual who needs to work on their well-being: Exercise, eat a fair eating routine, keep a solid weight, get great rest, lessen pressure, keep away from tobacco, and cutoff how much liquor you drink.

However, for disease survivors, the accompanying methodologies have added benefits. These straightforward advances can work on your satisfaction, smoothing your change into survivorship. This is how you might deal with yourself after malignant growth treatment.

1. Work out: Customary activity expands your feeling of prosperity after disease treatment and can speed your recuperation.

Disease survivors who exercise might have insight:

- Expanded strength and perseverance
- fewer signs and side effects of wretchedness
- Less nervousness
- Diminished exhaustion
- Further developed mindset
- Higher confidence

• Less agony

• Further developed rest

• Lower chance of the disease repeating

Adding actual work to your day-to-day schedule doesn't take a ton of additional work. Center around little moves toward making your life more dynamic. Use the stairwell more regularly or park farther from your objective and walk the remainder of the way. Check with your primary care physician before you start any activity program.

With your PCP's endorsement, begin gradually and move gradually up. The American Cancer Society suggests grown-up disease survivors practice for no less than 150 minutes per week, including strength preparing something like two days every week. As you recuperate and change, you could find that more activity causes you to feel quite a bit improved.

Some of the time you won't want to exercise, and that is OK. Try not to feel regretful if waiting for treatment aftereffects, for example, weakness, keep you sidelined. At the point when you feel like it, go for a stroll around the block. Give your best, and recall that rest additionally means quite a bit to your recuperation.

The practice has many advantages, and a few early examinations recommended that it might likewise diminish the gamble of a disease repeating and lessen the gamble of passing on from malignant growth. Numerous malignant growth survivors are worried about disease repeat and maintain that should give their best to stay away from it.

While the proof that exercise can decrease the gamble of passing on from disease is a starter, the proof of the advantages of activity to your heart, lungs and other body frameworks are significant. Thus, malignant growth survivors are urged to work out.

2. Eat a reasonable eating regimen: Change your eating regimen to incorporate bunches of foods grown from the ground, as well as entire grains. With regards to choosing your courses, the American Cancer Society suggests that disease survivors:

• Eat somewhere around 2.5 cups of products of the soil consistently

• Pick solid fats, including omega-3 unsaturated fats, like those tracked down in fish and pecans

· Select proteins that are low in soaked fat, like fish, lean meats, eggs, nuts, seeds, and vegetables

· Pick solid wellsprings of carbs, like entire grains, vegetables, and foods grown from the ground

This mix of food varieties will guarantee that you're eating a lot of the nutrients and supplements you want to assist with making your body solid.

It's not known whether a specific eating routine or certain supplements can hold malignant growth back from repeating. Concentrates on looking at low-fat eating regimens or diets that contain explicit products of the soil have had blended results. By and large, it's smart to eat a shifted diet that underlines products of the soil.

While enhancing your eating routine with a large group of nutrient and mineral enhancements, oppose that urge might entice. Some disease survivors feel that if a modest quantity of nutrients is great, a huge sum should be far superior. Yet, that isn't true. A lot of specific supplements can hurt you, truth be told.

On the off chance that you're worried about getting every one of the nutrients you want, inquire as to whether taking a day-to-day multivitamin is ideal for you.

3. Keep a solid weight: You might have acquired or shed pounds during treatment. Attempt to get your weight to a sound level. Converse with your primary care physician about what a sound weight is for yourself and the most effective way to approach accomplishing that objective weight.

For disease survivors who need to put on weight, this will probably include thinking of ways of making food engaging and simpler to eat. Converse with a dietitian who can assist you with formulating ways of putting on weight securely.

You and your primary care physician can cooperate to control sickness, torment, or opposite symptoms of malignant growth therapy that might be keeping you from getting the sustenance you want.

For disease survivors who need to get thinner, do whatever it takes to get in shape gradually — something like 2 pounds (around 1 kilogram) seven days.

Control the number of calories you eat and offset this with work out. On the off chance that you want to lose a great deal of weight, it can appear to be overwhelming. Take it gradually and stick to it.

4. Rest well: Rest issues are more normal in individuals with the disease, even survivors. This can be because of actual changes, results of treatment, stress, or different reasons.

Be that as it may, getting sufficient rest is a significant piece of your recuperation. Resting gives your psyche and body time to restore and revive to assist you with working at your best while you're alert. Getting great rest can support mental abilities, further develop chemical capability, and lower circulatory strain. It can likewise cheer you up overall.

To advance your opportunities to get great rest, practice solid rest cleanliness:

- Stay away from caffeine for no less than 8 hours before sleep time
- Adhere to a customary rest plan
- Stay away from PC or TV evaluates for 1 to 2 hours before sleep time
- Practice no later than 2 to 3 hours before hitting the hay
- Keep your room peaceful and faint

Assuming you feel unreasonably tired during the day, talk with your primary care physician. You might have a rest issue or an issue brought about by symptoms of your disease or its treatment.

5. Diminish pressure: As a malignant growth survivor, you might find that the physical, close-to-home, and social impacts have negatively affected your mind. However, no proof overseeing pressure further develops chances of malignant growth endurance, utilizing compelling survival methods to manage pressure can enormously work on your satisfaction by easing gloom, tension, and side effects connected with the disease and its treatment.

Compelling pressure the executive's techniques might include:

- Unwinding or reflection methods, for example, care preparing
- Directing
- Malignant growth support gatherings
- Prescriptions for sorrow or tension
- Work out

· Connecting with loved ones

6. Quit utilizing tobacco: Phase out the vice for the last time. Smoking or utilizing biting tobacco seriously endangers you of a few kinds of disease. Halting now could diminish your gamble of malignant growth repeating and bring down your gamble of fostering the second sort of disease (second essential malignant growth).

If you've taken a stab at stopping before but haven't had a lot of progress, look for help. Converse with your primary care physician about assets to assist you with stopping.

7. Savor liquor control, if by any stretch of the imagination: Assuming you decide to drink liquor, do as such with some restraint. For sound grown-ups, that implies dependent upon one beverage daily for ladies of any age and men more established than age 65, and up to two beverages every day for men age 65 and more youthful.

Liquor has medical advantages for certain individuals — for example, polishing off a beverage daily can lessen your gamble of coronary illness. In any case, it likewise builds the gamble of specific diseases, including those of the mouth and throat.

While it isn't evident whether drinking liquor can cause disease to repeat, it can build your gamble of a second essential malignant growth.

Gauge the dangers and advantages of drinking liquor and talk it over with your primary care physician.

Conclusion

The standpoint for an individual getting chemotherapy will rely to a great extent upon the sort, stage, and area of the malignant growth and an individual's general wellbeing. At times, the complete reduction is conceivable.

There can be unfavorable impacts, notwithstanding, and individuals might have to change their way of life or work routine during treatment. Notwithstanding, these generally resolve after treatment wraps up.

Before beginning treatment, an individual might wish to examine with the specialist:

- why do they are suggesting chemotherapy
- what different choices are
- which kinds of chemotherapy are accessible
- the amount it will cost
- what's in store concerning unfriendly impacts

They may likewise need to contact:

- a protection supplier about taking care of the expenses
- their boss, if pertinent, about what treatment might mean for their work schedule
- family, companions, or guardians about what's in store

A specialist can frequently place an individual in contact with a guide or care group, who might help.